HEALTHY HABITS
WITH OR WITHOUT DIABETES

written by
FLOYD STOKES

illustrated by
SHEENA HISIRO

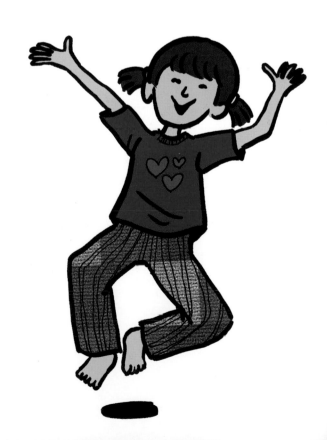

Brought to you by

PINNACLEHEALTH
Auxiliary

PinnacleHealth Auxiliary
Mission Statement

The PinnacleHealth Auxiliary is a volunteer community organization dedicated to supporting PinnacleHealth System in its endeavors to provide quality healthcare and health education in Central Pennsylvania.

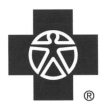

Capital BlueCross
Independent Licensee of the BlueCross BlueShield Association

Capital BlueCross is celebrating 75 years of improving the health and well-being of the men, women and children in central Pennsylvania and the Lehigh Valley.

A publication of the American Literacy Corporation for Young Readers

Text copyright © 2012 by Floyd Stokes.
Illustrations copyright © 2013 by Sheena Hisiro.
Graphic Design by Sheena Hisiro.
First Edition, 2013. All rights reserved.

ISBN 978-0-9797871-4-0

PRINTED IN CHINA

Special thanks to the members of
Pinnacle Health Auxiliary and Capital
Blue Cross team who helped to develop
the book. Your input was invaluable.

f.s.

To Rachael-
s.h.

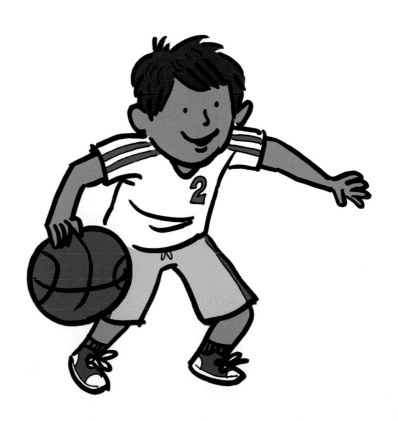

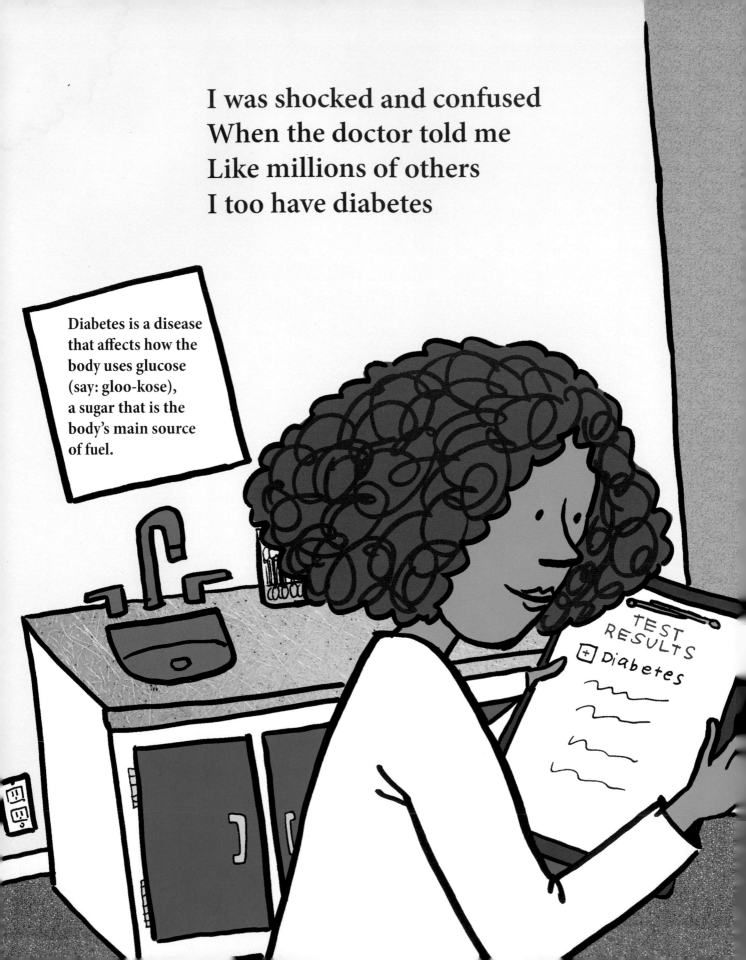

I thought it was a disease
For only adults
Until the doctor gave me
My test results

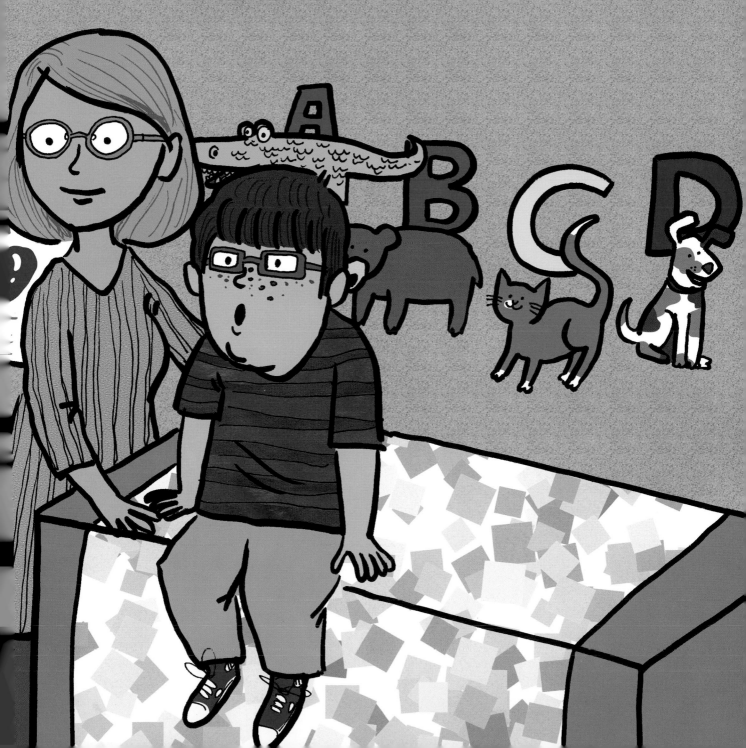

I have diabetes, but others can't catch it
I can reduce the effects by staying active and fit
There is no cure but I can manage it
By making healthy choices about my diet

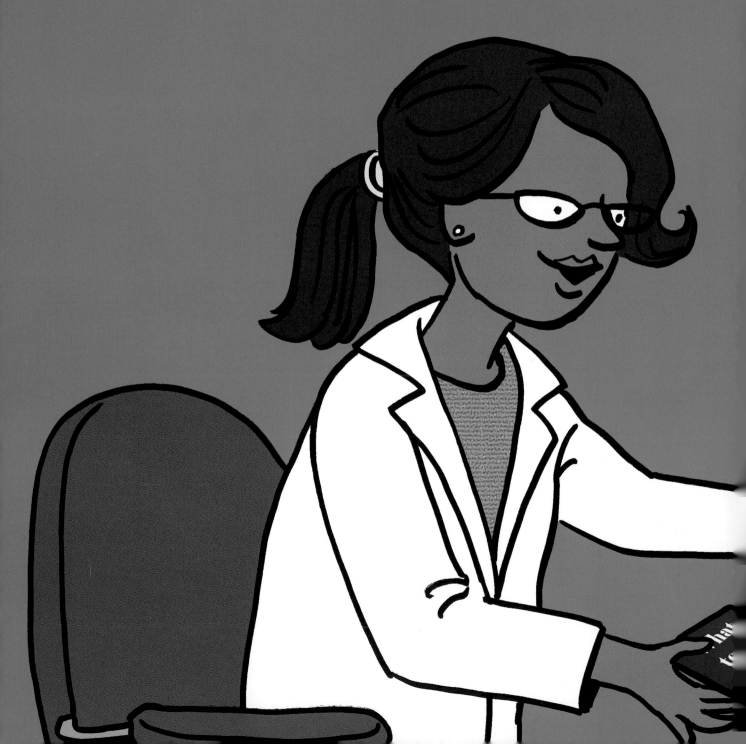

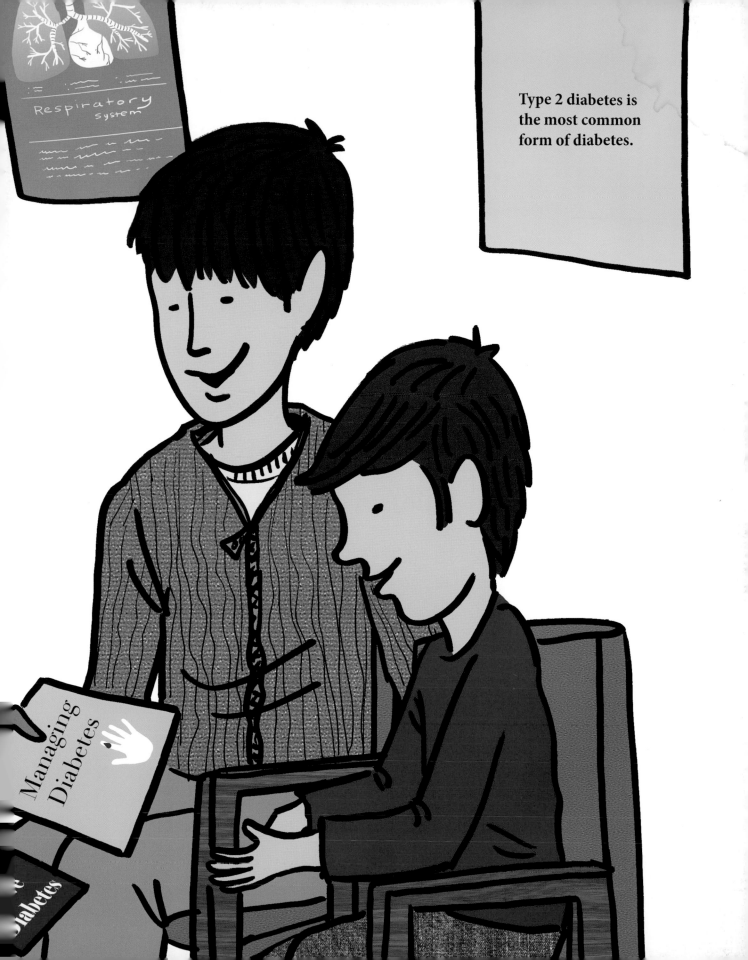

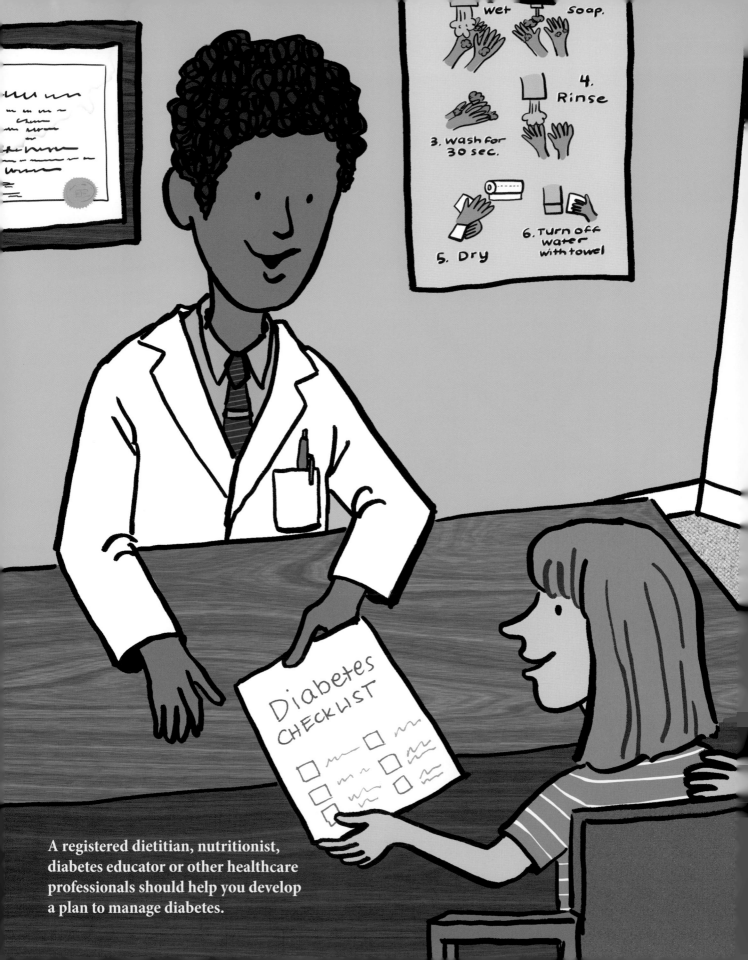

A registered dietitian, nutritionist, diabetes educator or other healthcare professionals should help you develop a plan to manage diabetes.

The doctor and I
Came up with a plan
At first I wasn't sure
But now, I know I can

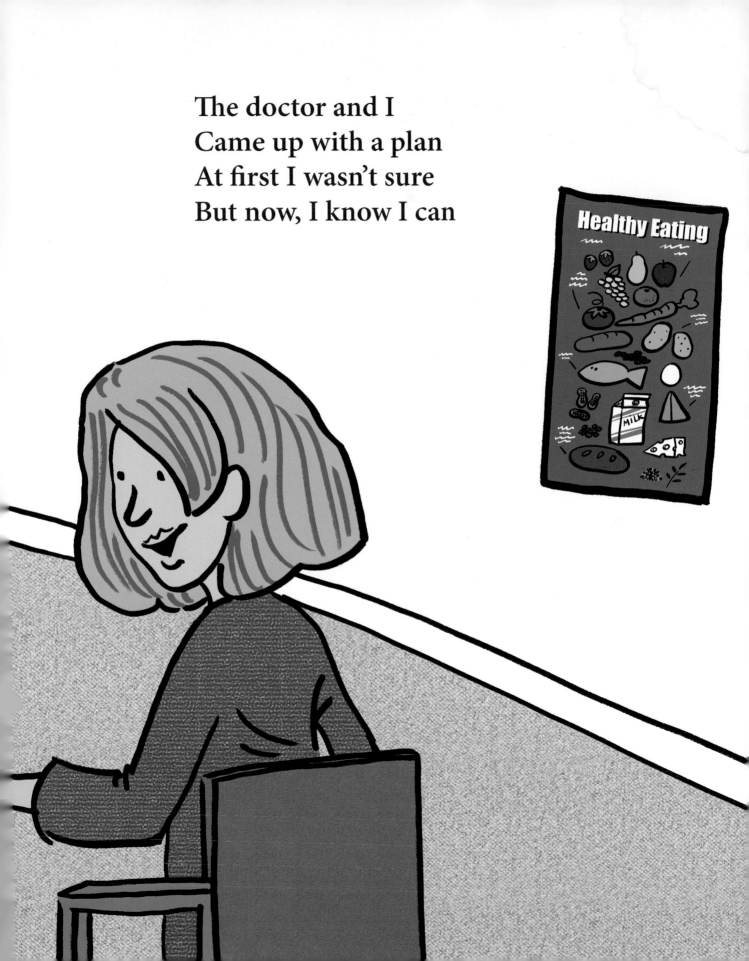

He told me to relax

To improve my mood

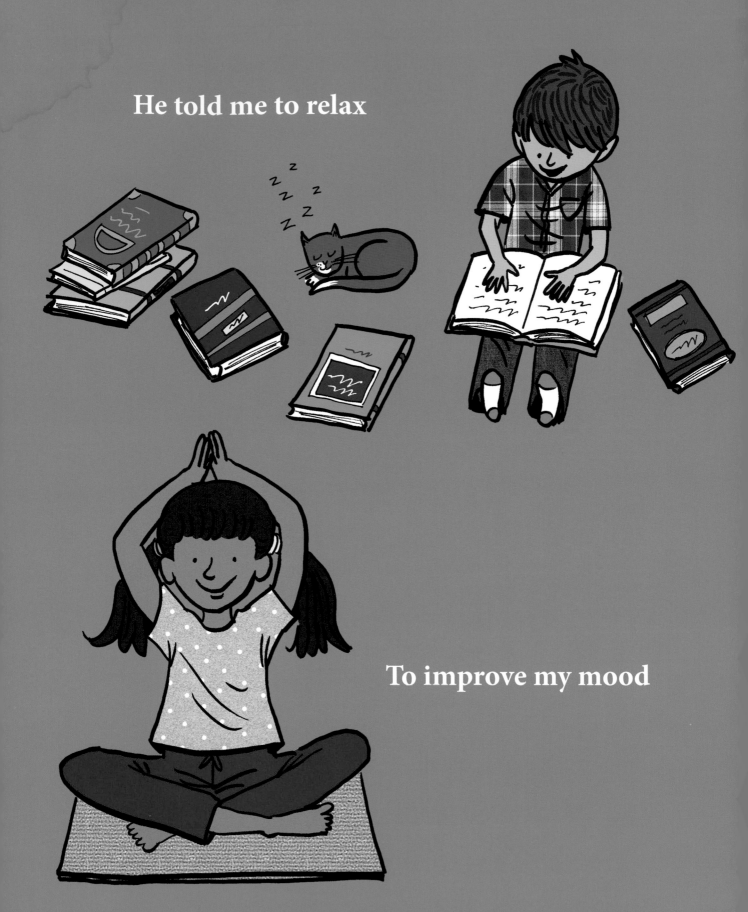

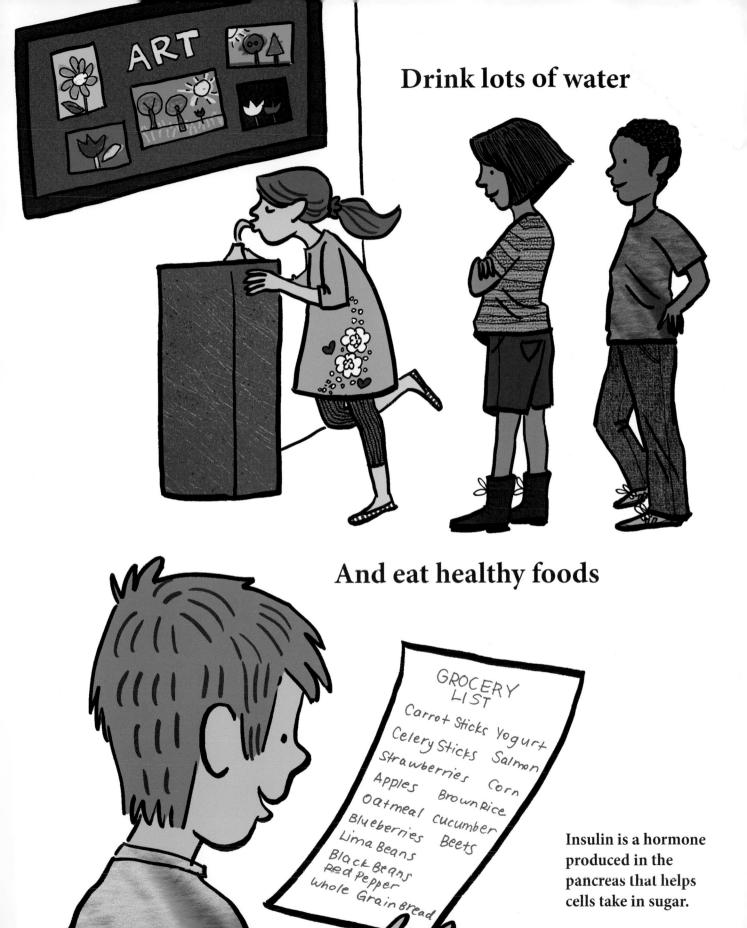

Drink lots of water

And eat healthy foods

GROCERY LIST

Carrot Sticks   Yogurt
Celery Sticks   Salmon
Strawberries   Corn
Apples   Brown Rice
Oatmeal   Cucumber
Blueberries   Beets
Lima Beans
Black Beans
Red Pepper
Whole Grain Bread

Insulin is a hormone produced in the pancreas that helps cells take in sugar.

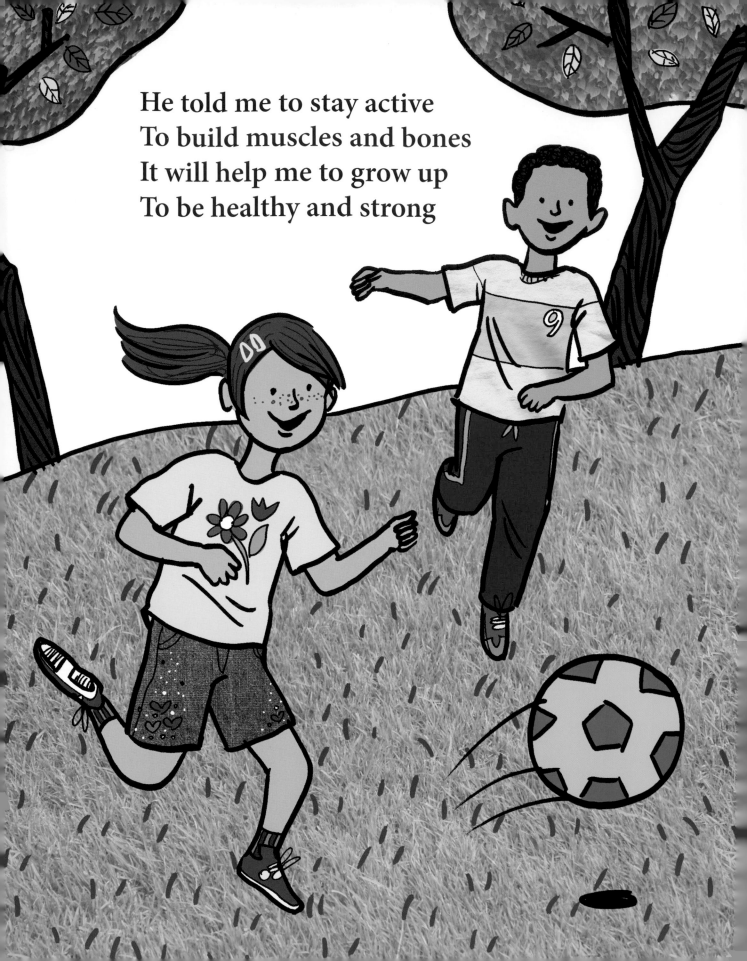

He told me to stay active
To build muscles and bones
It will help me to grow up
To be healthy and strong

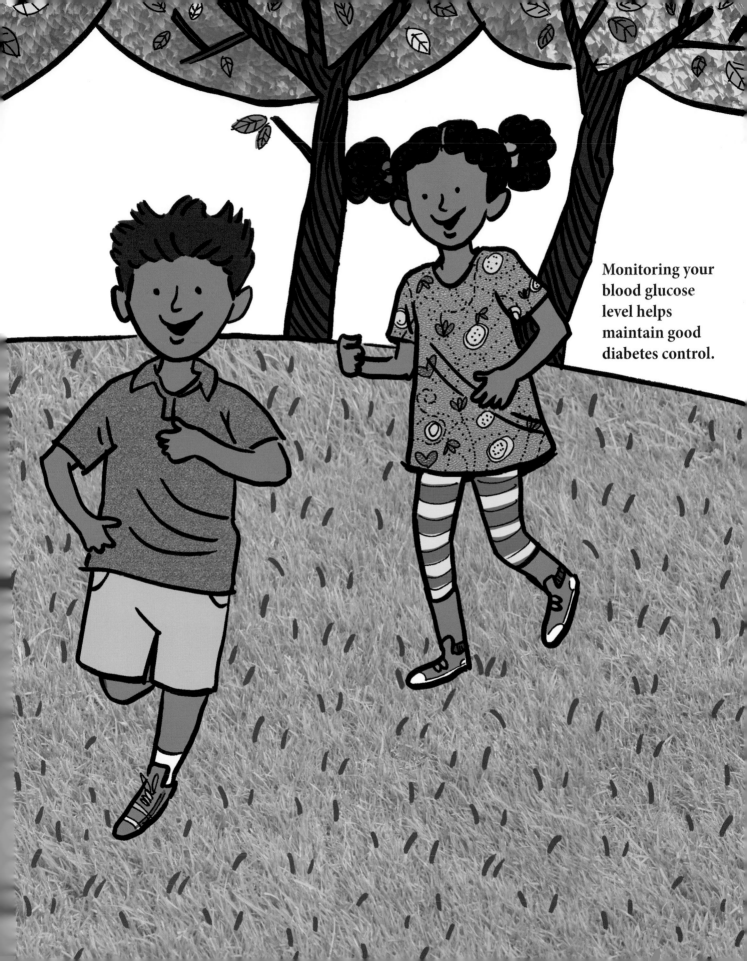

Monitoring your blood glucose level helps maintain good diabetes control.

I stay active and fit throughout the day
Whether at home, school or at play

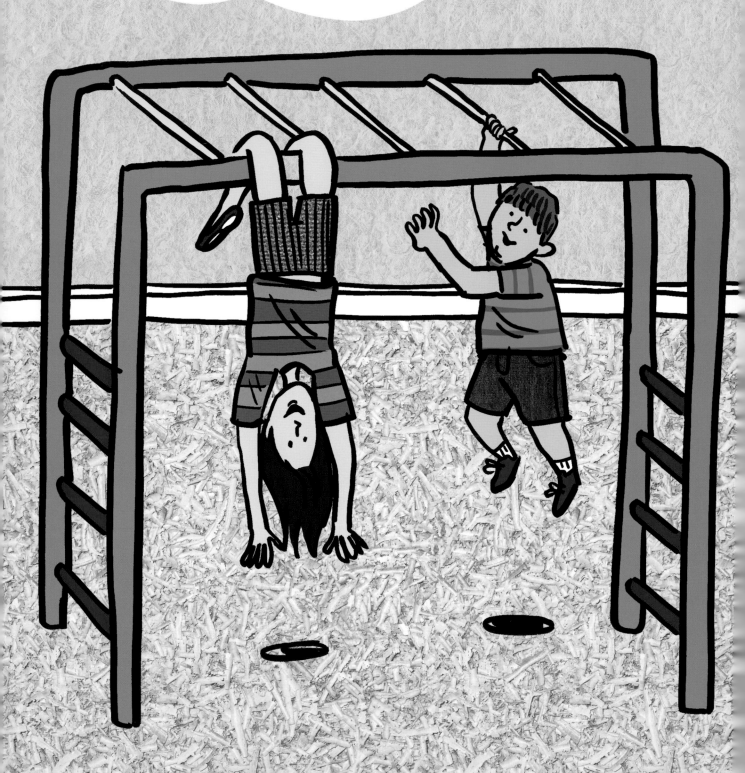

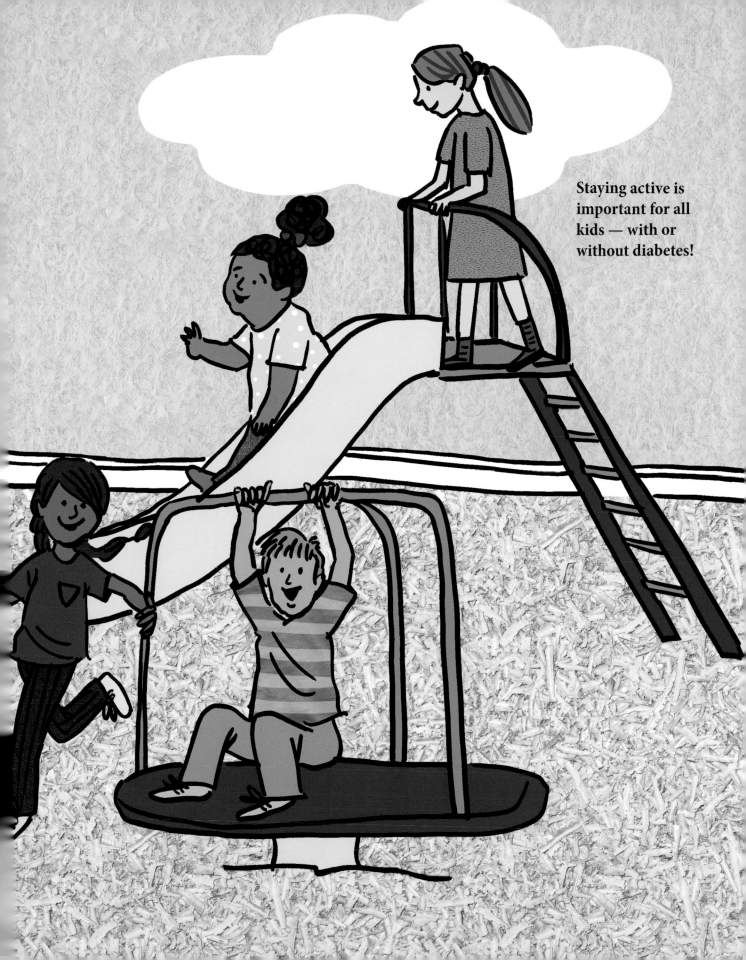

Staying active is important for all kids — with or without diabetes!

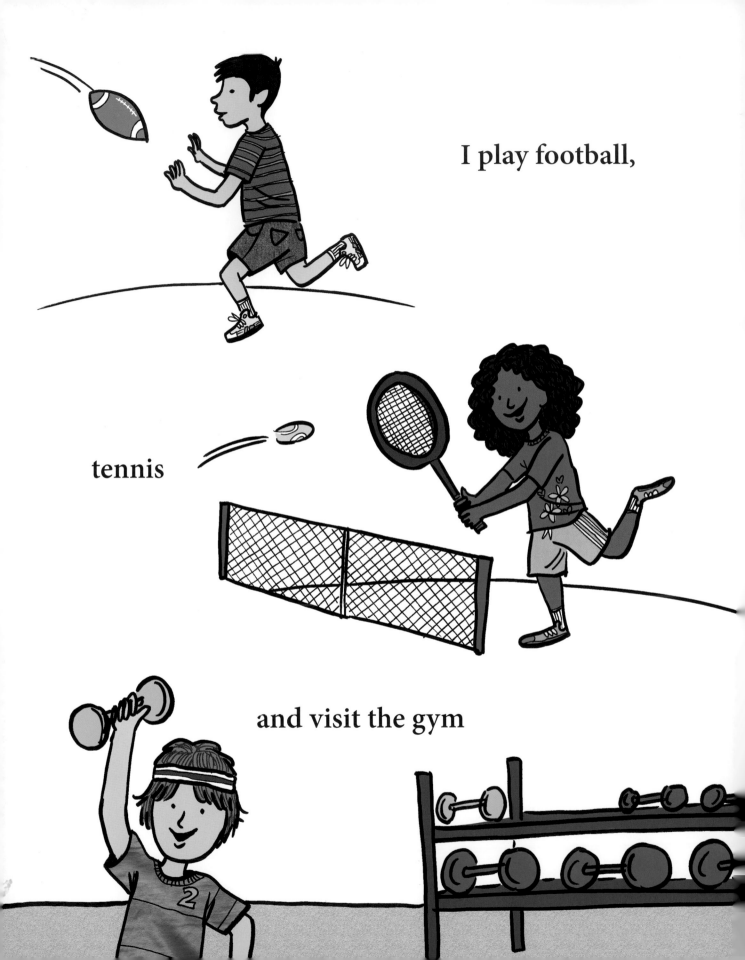

I play football,

tennis

and visit the gym

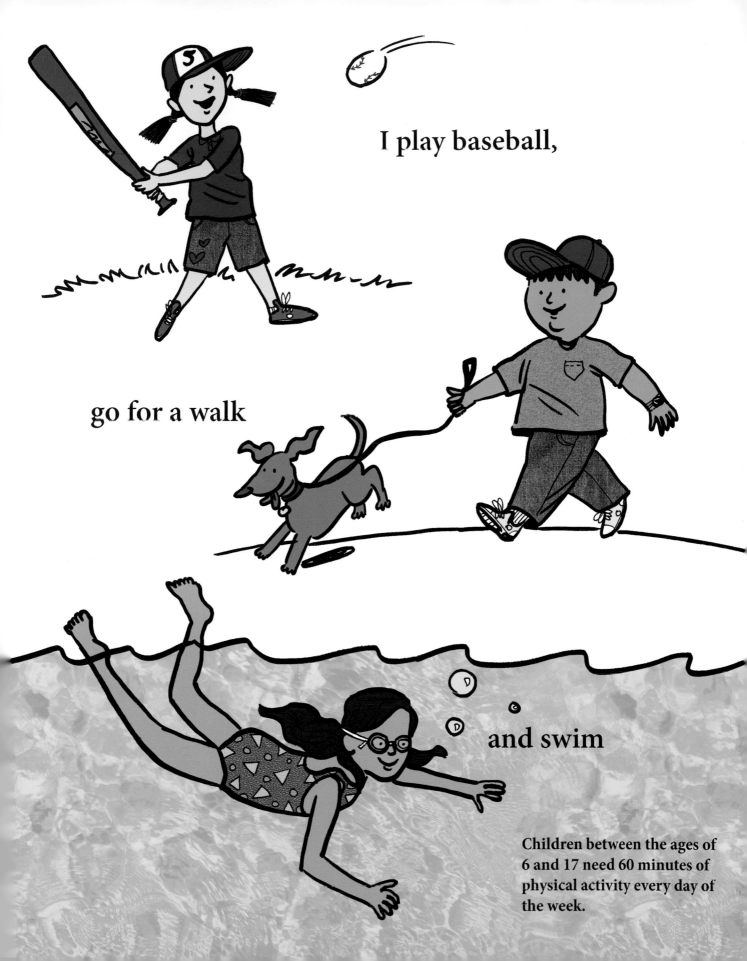

I play baseball,

go for a walk

and swim

Children between the ages of 6 and 17 need 60 minutes of physical activity every day of the week.

I learned to eat the food I need
A balanced diet will help me succeed

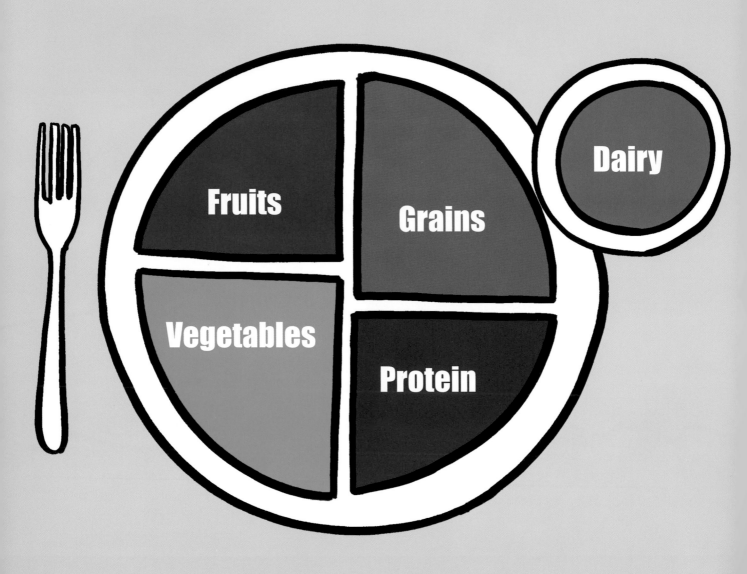

**A healthy diet is the same
for everyone, whether or
not you have diabetes.**

I reduced the amount of fat I eat
I replaced it with fish and lean meat

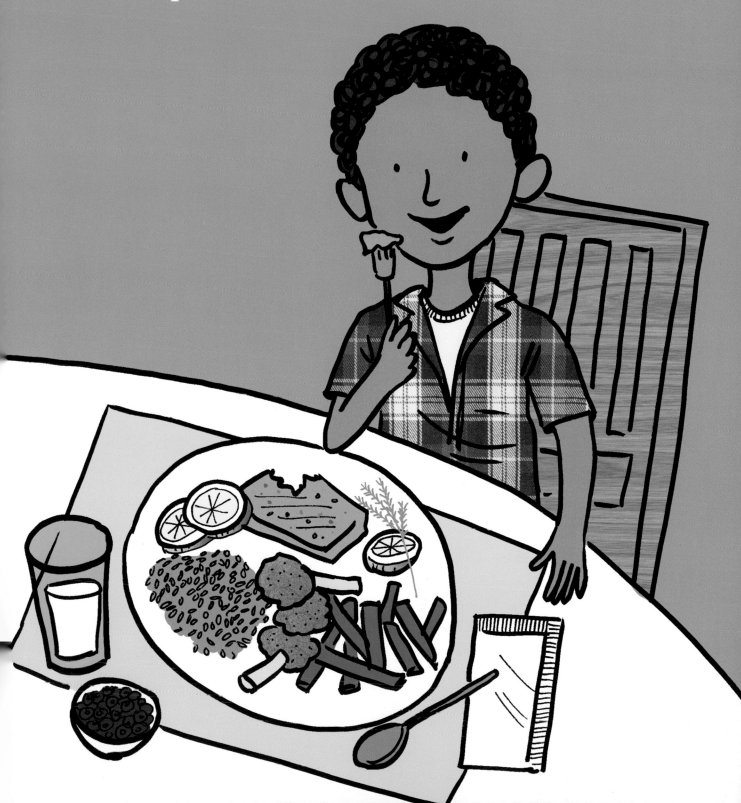

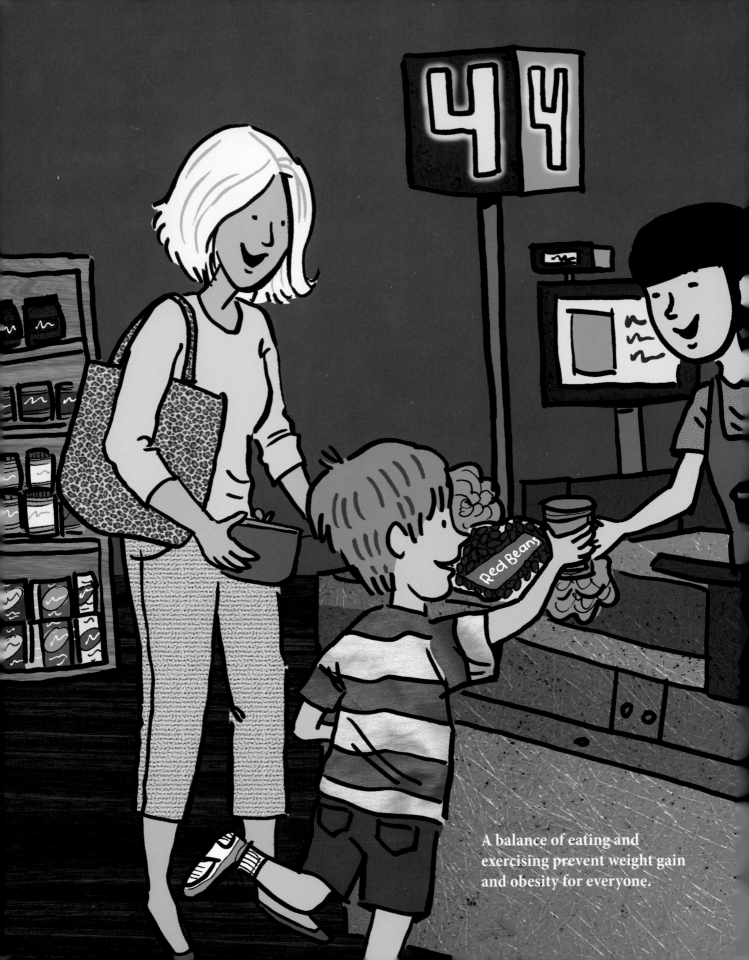

A balance of eating and exercising prevent weight gain and obesity for everyone.

I eat lettuce, cucumbers, beans and beets
Corn, oatmeal and bread that's whole wheat

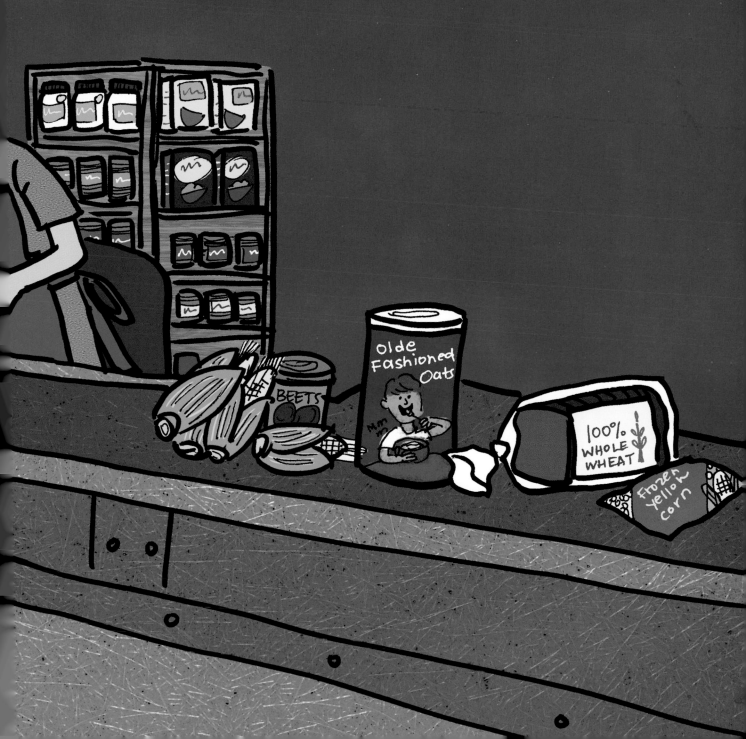

I reduced chips and candy, soda and cake
Instead of fried, I eat chicken that's baked

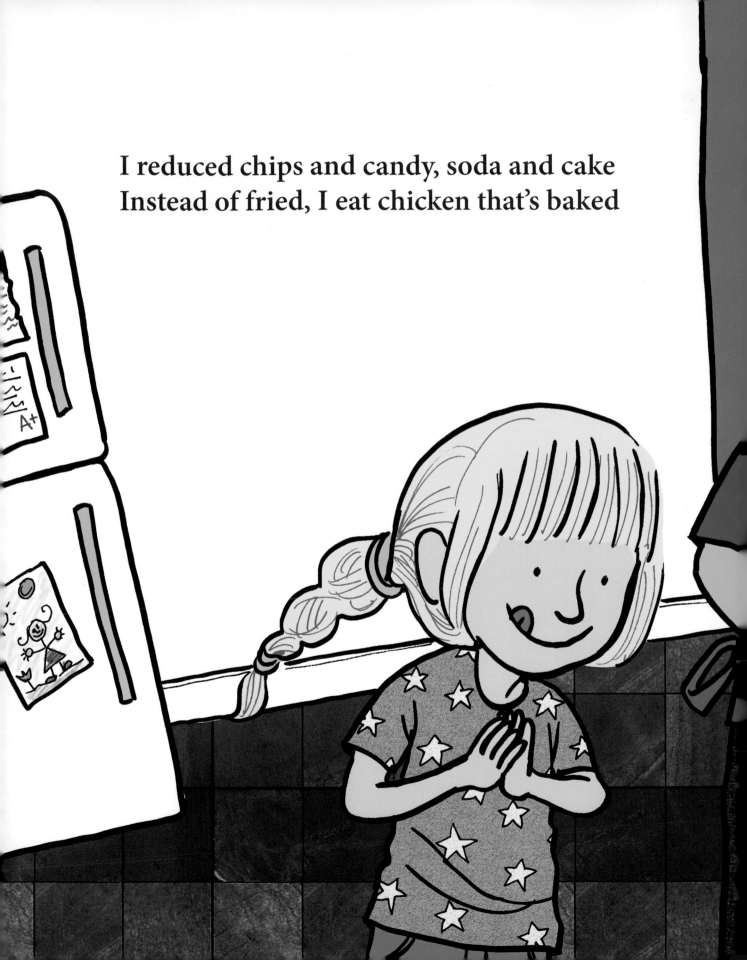

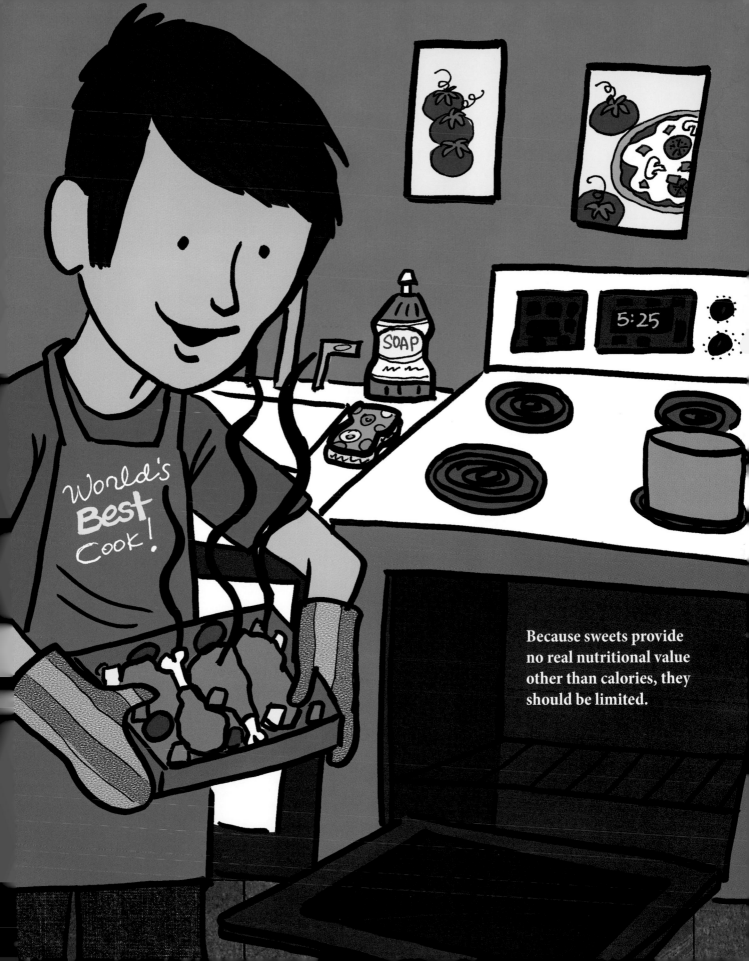

Because sweets provide no real nutritional value other than calories, they should be limited.

I eat super foods like spinach and greens
And lima, black, and pinto beans
Grilled, roasted, baked or steamed
It makes me healthy and boosts my esteem

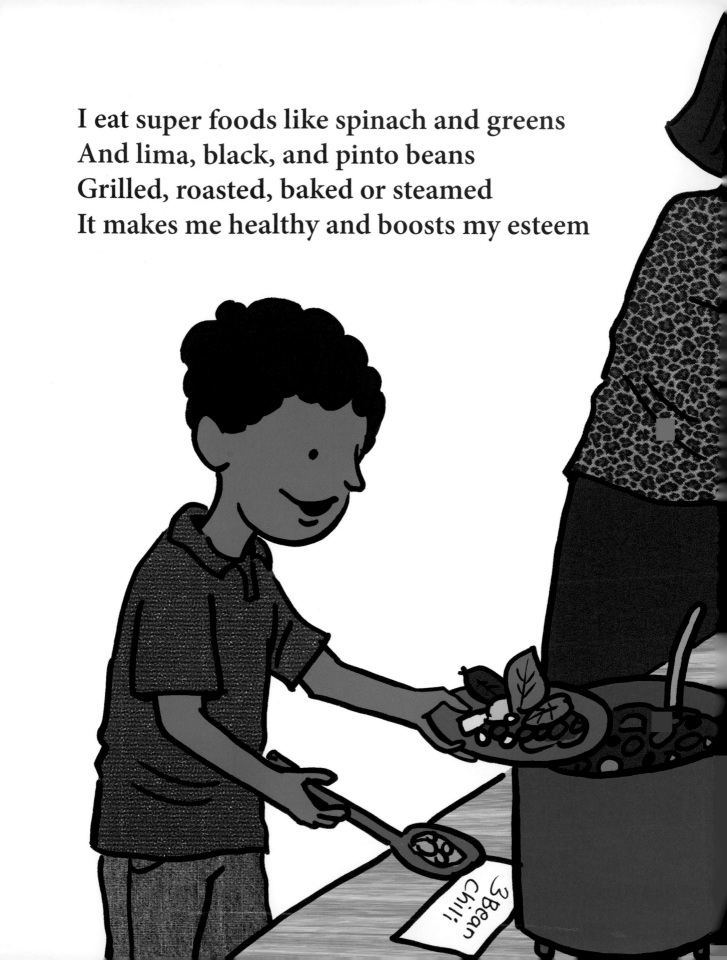

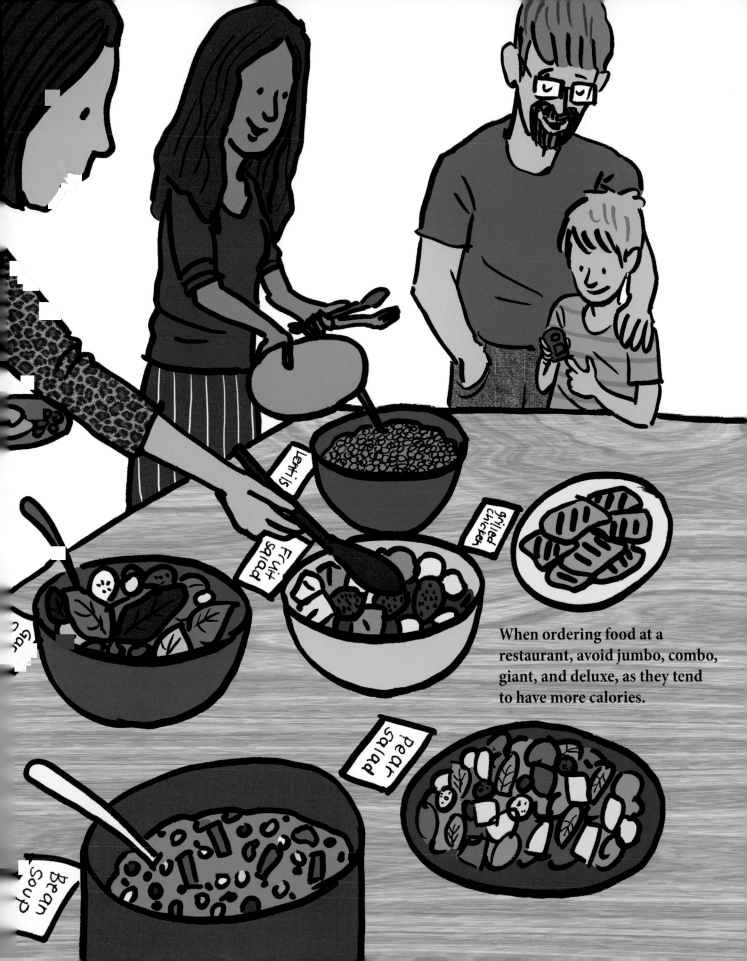

When ordering food at a restaurant, avoid jumbo, combo, giant, and deluxe, as they tend to have more calories.

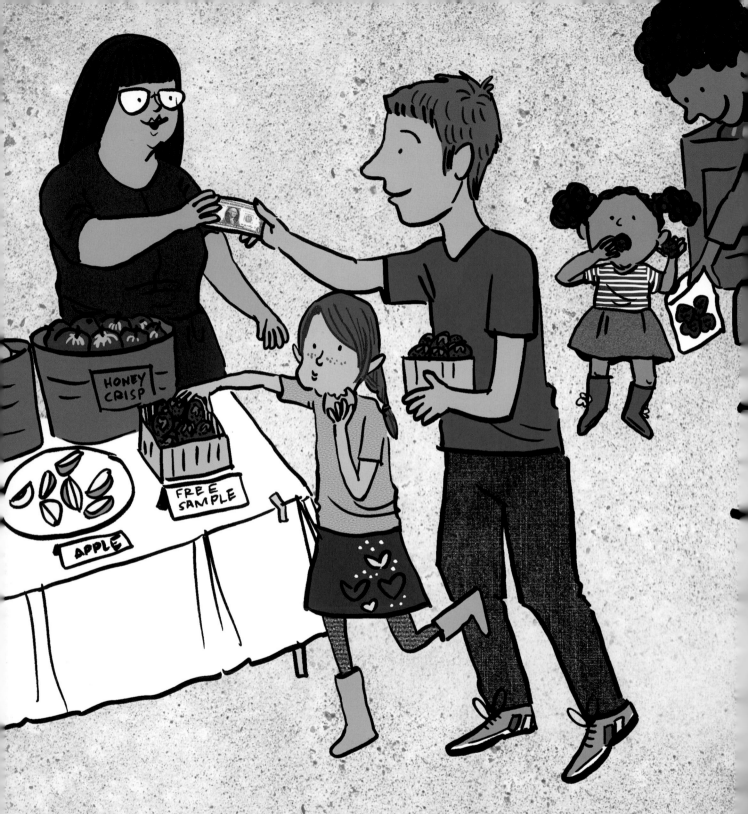

I eat apples, bananas and grapes for a snack
Watermelon and berries red and black

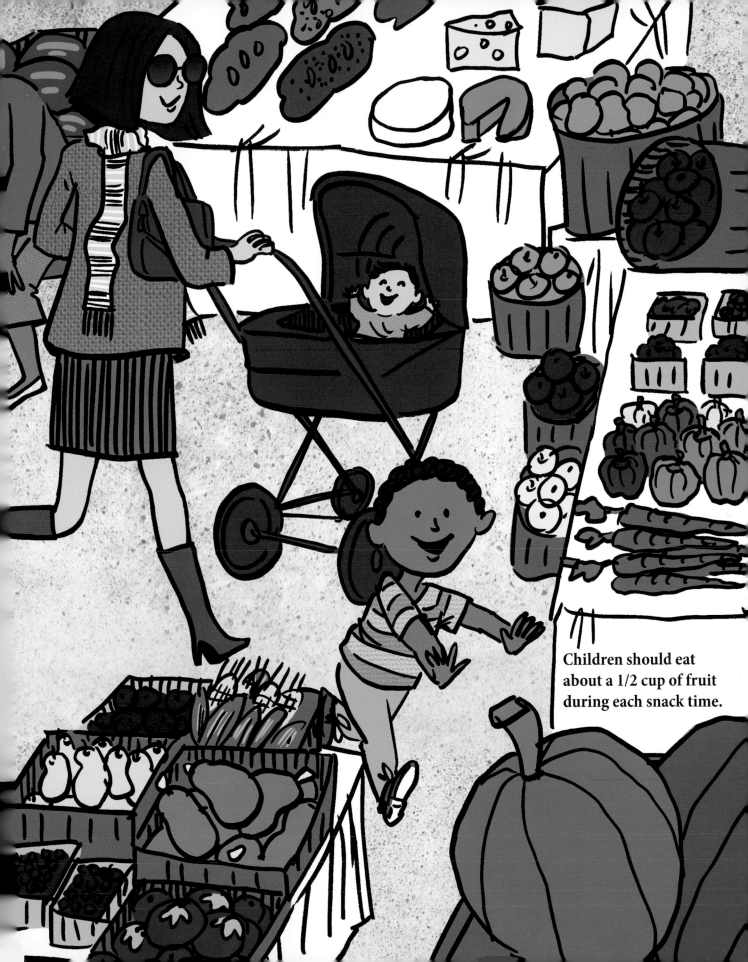

Children should eat about a 1/2 cup of fruit during each snack time.

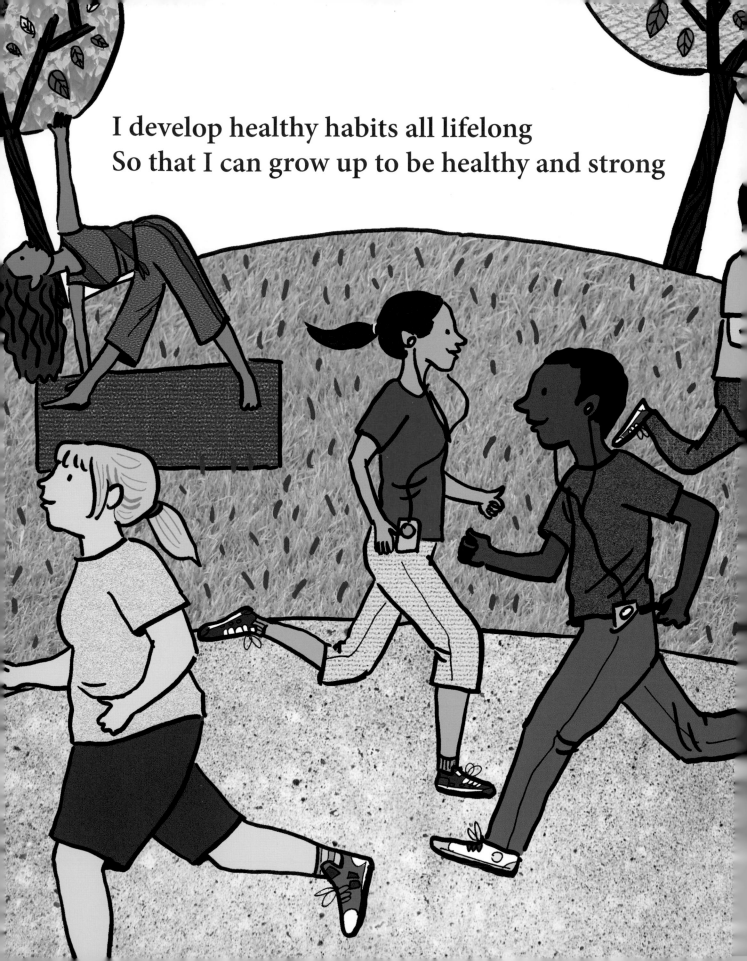

I develop healthy habits all lifelong
So that I can grow up to be healthy and strong

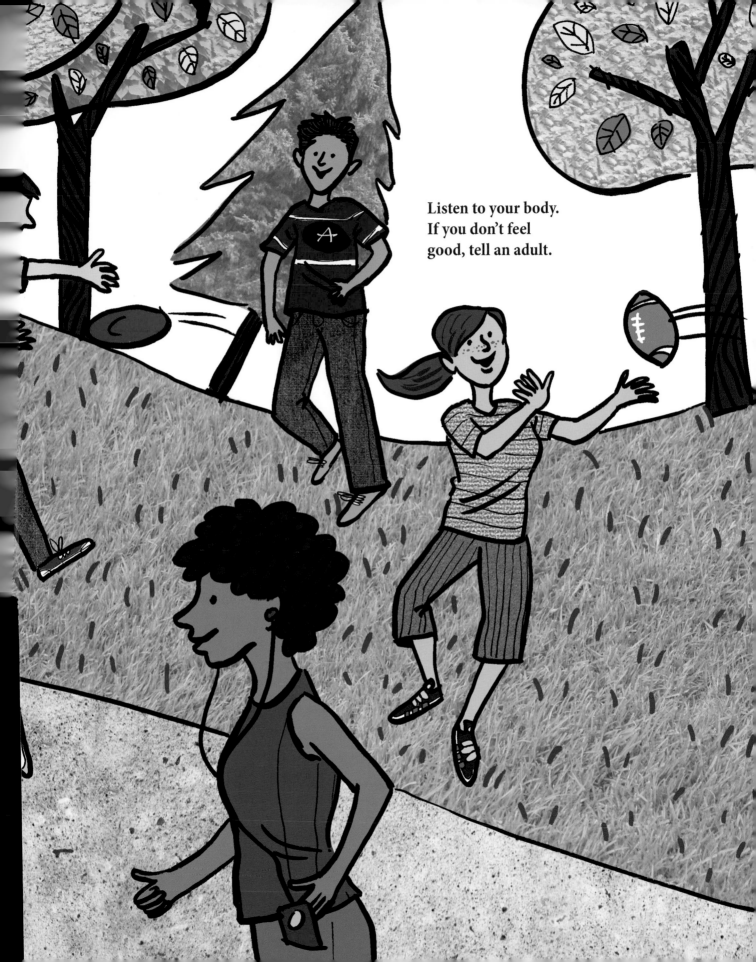

Listen to your body.
If you don't feel
good, tell an adult.

THE DIGESTIVE SYSTEM

When you eat food, the body breaks down all of the sugars and starches into glucose, which is the basic fuel for the cells in the body. Below are basic organs associated with the digestive system.

Esophagus - is a muscular tube which carries food and liquids from the throat to the stomach.

Thoracic diaphragm - is a sheet of internal skeletal muscle that extends across the bottom of the rib cage.

Stomach - is an organ between the esophagus and the small intestine. It is where digestion of food begins.

Liver - a large reddish brown organ in vertebrates that secretes bile and cleanses the blood and is located in the abdominal cavity.

Spleen - is a ductless organ that filters and stores blood, destroys certain worn-out red blood cells, and produces certain white blood cells of the immune system.

Gallbladder - is a small organ that aids mainly in fat digestion and concentrates bile produced by the liver.

Duodenum - is the first section of the small intestine.

Pancreas – is a gland located near the stomach that secretes a digestive juice into the intestine and insulin into the blood.

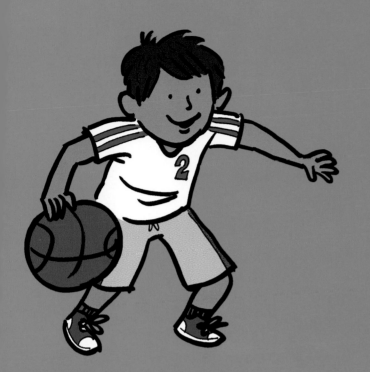
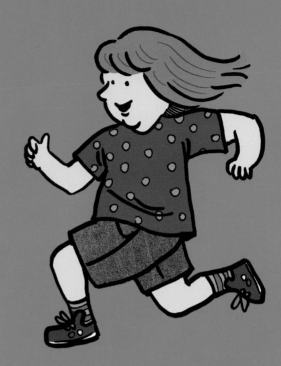

Could you have Diabetes?
Below are the common warning signs:

- Thirst
- Excessive urination
- Extreme Fatigue
- Blurred vision
- Delayed healing of wounds
- Skin infections
- Change in Weight

From www.pinnaclehealth.org/diabetes

Some of the facts in this book were from the following websites.
http://www.dosomething.org/tipsandtools/11-facts-about-diabetes-children
http://www.diabetes.org/diabetes-basics/type-2/

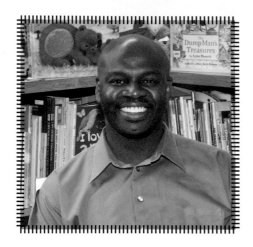

FLOYD STOKES is the founder and Executive Director of the American Literacy Corporation (ALC). He has written 11 books to include: *Say Ahh! The Teeth Book, Popcorn, There Was an Old Lady Who Lived in a Shoe, My Glasses, Bullying is BAD,* and *AJ the Rooster*. On May 1, 2009, he was awarded an honorary doctorate of humanities from Central Penn College. In 2010, he read to children in all 50 states.

For more info, visit:
www.superreader.org

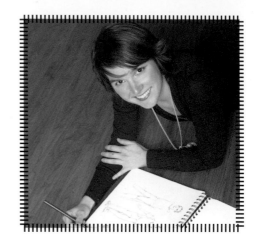

SHEENA HISIRO has been drawing since she could hold a pencil. She currently lives in Brooklyn, NY, where she is still drawing and loving every minute of it. Sheena has a BFA in Communications Design from Pratt Institute. She has illustrated 12 other books including *The Boy Who Cried Wolf!, My Glasses, Bullying is BAD, I Can Do It By Myself,* and *Josiah and Julia Go to Church*.

For more info, visit:
oodlesofdoodles.tumblr.com